And Then...Came Arthur
Hope Comes in Many Forms

Jennifer Thie

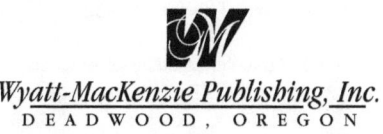

Wyatt-MacKenzie Publishing, Inc.
DEADWOOD, OREGON

And Then...Came Arthur: Hope Comes in Many Forms
by Jennifer Thie

ISBN-13: 978-1-932279-57-3

Library of Congress Control Number: 2007923475

© 2007 by Jennifer Thie. All Rights Reserved.

No part of this publication may be translated, reproduced or transmitted in any form or by any means, in whole or in part, without prior permission in writing from the publisher.

Publisher and editor are not liable for any typographical errors, content mistakes, inaccuracies, or omissions related to the information in this book.

Product trade names or trademarks mentioned throughout this publication remain property of their respective owners.

Wyatt-MacKenzie Publishing, Inc., Deadwood, OR
www.WyMacPublishing.com (541) 964-3314

Requests for permission or further information should be addressed to:
Wyatt-MacKenzie Publishing, 15115 Highway 36,
Deadwood, Oregon 97430

Printed in the United States of America

To my wonderful husband who makes me smile each and every day.

Table of Contents

Acknowledgments   7

Introduction   9

Chapter One: The Decision That Changed Our Lives   11

Chapter Two: Mom   15

Chapter Three: Being Pregnant   23

   Is Mine a Normal Pregnancy?   23

   Bed Rest? Not Me!   24

   Barely Room Enough   25

   One Big Happy Family   26

   Growing Larger as Time Grows Short   29

Chapter Four: Then the World Shuddered   31

   Empty Spaces   33

Chapter Five: Welcome New Souls!   37

   Help!   37

   Arrival   38

   Chapter Six: Complications   41

   Welcome Home   41

   Illness Strikes in Threes   42

Chapter Seven: Losing Mom   45

   Rushing   47

Fearful of the Worst   48

   Can It Get Worse?   50

   The Waiting Game   51

Chapter Eight: Dad   57

   Immigrants   58

   Best of Both Parents   63

   Growing Up with Dad   65

   Room to Grow Up   67

Chapter Nine: And Then Came Arthur   71

Chapter Ten: Where There's a Will, There's a Way   77

   Slowly Awakening   79

   Recovery   81

Chapter Eleven: Can Anything More Really Happen?   85

   Treatment   88

   More Drama   91

Chapter Twelve: The Fighting Spirit   95

Chapter Thirteen: Blessed   101

Acknowledgments

Many people made my life and this book possible.

Thank you Mom and Dad for being amazing parents and outstanding role models. I love you both so much. Thanks Bink for always standing by me no matter how high I let my "freak flag fly." Kathleen—you, Q & M mean the world to me. To my amazing Grandmothers, Mary (who I miss everyday) & Kathrine: I am so blessed to have had the love of these two strong woman. Paul and Marylou, thanks for all of your support. I do not know how we would have survived that first week without you. For my inner circle of goddesses, the best girlfriends in the whole world—Mills, Mer, Carol, Jarv and Sarah—you ladies are my touchstones. Thanks to all of the doctors, nurses, family and friends who touched my life and helped me through some very hard times. Each day I feel truly fortunate to live in our wonderful neighborhood of College Terrace; a place were myself and my family has developed life long friendships with some remarkable people. And to the late Dr. Donald Jordan who always could see my ability, not my disability. You were more then my college adviser, you were my friend. Thank you.

Dr. Caron Goode understood my vision, compassion and convictions. Her editing and assistance made this book come to life. Thank you, Caron. Nancy Cleary of Wyatt-MacKenzie Publishing made my dream to publish come true as she has for so many other women; your hard work and enthusiasm are truly amazing.

Finally, I need to acknowledge my little angels, my children. You are what make my life complete. I love you more than any words can express.

Introduction

When you are in the middle of an earthquake, you know the ground is shaking, but you can only hang on and pray to get through it. This story explores the nature of human spirituality in the face of the earthquakes in life known as birth, illness and death.

I started writing about my experiences as a mother after the birth of my beautiful boy/girl twins. As I shared my story with the local Mothers of Multiples chapter, the reality of what I had survived, before and after their birth, hit me like an aftershock.

My deepest desire is that you walk away from this book with a sense of hope and inspiration, fully appreciating the struggles you've conquered. Hope crept into the people in my life in small ways: my despondent dad's love of a feral dog; my comatose mom's request to listen to Howard Stern; me dragging myself out of bed during chemotherapy to hug my children.

My search for what makes some people strong and full of hope and spirituality took me to past generations. Here I saw my relatives approach religion in all sorts of ways—with deep formal conviction, with mixed feelings and with absolute rejection. Seeing all of this within my own family tree forced me to examine the question that has always tugged at me: What is required for one to be good and blessed?

In the end, I believe that it is what we think, say and do throughout life, and in the face of adversity, that determines whether we are good and blessed. Be a person of blessings; go about each and every day striving to be kind, good and truthful. Whether you do this on a large scale or in a small way, this is what makes you a blessed person.

Jennifer Thie
Winter, 2006

Chapter One

The Decision That Changed Our Lives

It was the tiniest thing I ever decided to put my whole life into. ~ Terri Guillemets

Robert and I were only moments away from the last step in the in-vitro fertilization procedure. For the last several months, my husband held my hand each step of the way through doctor's visits, shots and blood tests. Today, however, he decided to sit out this last procedure and read *Car & Driver* in the waiting room. Perhaps the stirrups on the exam table scared him away, but more than likely, the new issue of *Car & Driver* kept Robert from being witness to one of the life-altering moments in our marriage.

So I was alone in the stirrups when the doctor came in and said, "Well, I've got good news!"

"Oh yeah?" He had caught my interest.

"Jennifer, your embryos are so viable that if I put in two, I can almost guarantee that you and Robert will have twins."

"Sounds great." I blurted out those words so quickly, with no second thought about how two words would change two lives. Divine inspiration? Maybe?

I walked into the waiting room fifteen minutes later, grinning like the Cheshire Cat. "Robert, we are going to have twins."

He was speechless. His eyes widened and his mouth dropped open. His face expressed a combination of complete surprise, excitement, bewilderment and creeping primal fear.

"Robert" I reminded him, "if you had just come into the room with me for this last step, you might have had more input."

I wish I could say that Robert had some influence on this the most important decision of our lives, but he didn't. In reality, I had decided when we started the in-vitro fertilization (IVF) treatments that the idea of having twins sounded great. Presto! One pregnancy and I would be done. Who knows? I could even have a boy and a girl.

Have you heard women say that they knew the precise moment when they got pregnant? I was one of those women. Honestly, the very second the doctor inserted the two embryos within me I knew I was pregnant. Unlike so many women who have tried IVF repeatedly with one failed attempt after another, this was my first try. What a miracle!

My getting-pregnant problem had been those damn tubes. The doctor told me he had never seen anything like my perfectly flat fallopian tubes. No eggs, or sperm for that matter, were getting through those things. Was I born this way? Maybe. Or maybe my tubes were flattened by endless years of gymnastics. Did wrapping my hips around the bars over and over again flatten them like pancakes? I'll never know.

Our first plan of action was to reshape the tubes through surgery. After only a few months of trying to get pregnant after surgery, I threw in the towel and jumped into the fertility treatments. At thirty-one, I was one of the youngest women at University Hospital's Infertility Center.

Fertility treatments are big business in the Silicon Valley because so many women wait until after their careers to start their families. And who can blame them? Stock options increasing in value by the minute and the chance to become millionaires are very strong temptations. Who had time to get pregnant, let alone meet a mate?

I wasn't one of those women however. Before I finished college, I had a non-high-tech job in sales, working for my dad. Within several years, I was happily married to a non-high tech guy. We did not have the stock options, but we had good stable jobs, which not everyone in the San Francisco Bay Area could claim. The only thing that was missing in our world was a baby—or babies.

That was all about to change. As I walked out of the infertility clinic, my husband trailed behind me, still shaking his head in the haze of "What just happened?"

Chapter Two

Mom

Mother—that was the bank where we deposited all our hurts and worries.
~ DeWitt Talmage

Character contributes to beauty. It fortifies a woman as her youth fades. ~ Jacqueline Bisset

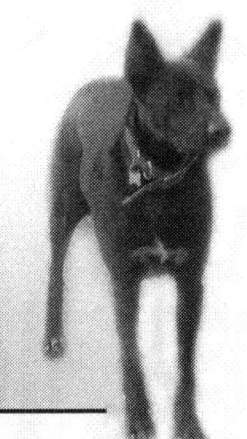

After the insemination, Robert and I visited my mother's office in the Cardiac Surgery Lab at University Hospital where Catherine had worked for the past twenty-four years.

My parents were twenty-one years old when they married. My brother came along less then 2 years after me. Mom put college on hold while she stayed home with me and my brother during those early years. When our family relocated to the San Francisco Bay Area from Los Angeles, my mom completed her Bachelor of Science degree and started working at the University Hospital where they provided flexible work hours.

Catherine started as a lab technician in the Cardiac Surgery Lab, researching the use of heart pumps when I was seven– years old. She worked nights and my father worked days to insure that that one would be home with my brother and me.

As her career progressed, Mom worked her way up the chain of command at the hospital, which was not easy to do without a doctoral degree. By the time I was in high school, she was managing the lab.

Because a cow's heart is similar to a human heart, Mom inserted heart pumps in the cows and cared for them in a very humane way. I sort back through my memories and think how perfect my mother was to work in a lab with animals to support human life and health. She loved animals, she had the greatest respect for their lives, and she also enjoyed and respected science.

Within the lab setting, mom didn't want animals to suffer, and she treated her animals with great regard. Her work is research for healing heart disease and she values human life as much as she does animal life. I thought this position spoke highly of her efforts and skills and she had a knack for this work. The irony of the situation is that my father, a vegetarian and animal lover for many years, rarely went to mother's place of work.

When the lab moved to new facilities, they switched from using cows to sheep because they did not grow as quickly and the lab now had longer data-gathering periods. One of the hardest parts of the research was keeping the animals alive after the insertion of the heart pump. In this area, my mother excelled. She had the most effective way of keeping cows, and later sheep, alive after their artificial heart pumps failed. She was able to keep the animals alive longer, I believe, because of her care giving.

When Catherine talked, people listened. Even doctors listened to her when it came to keeping animals alive in the cardiovascular lab. Like most animal lovers, I hated the idea of these poor animals dying in the name of some fat slob who ate, drank, and smoked himself into heart disease.

However, my mother would quickly remind me that her work was saving the lives of thousands of people who were born with congenital heart disease, not just the ones who may bring it on to themselves. She explained that her research had a purpose; it was not like she was working for a cosmetic company who was burning out the eyes of bunnies to make sure the lipstick would not come off five hours after putting it on.

By the time I was in middle school, Mom was extremely involved in her work. Regardless, she always made it a point to show up for my diving meets or gymnastics. I had lunch with her once a week at the hospital cafeteria. She would make sure that we ate at the Children's Hospital and always say, "The food is better over here, don't you think?"

No, I did not think that the food was better; it was the same crappy food that they served in the main part of the hospital. The only difference was the cafeteria at Children's Hospital was full of sick children and grieving families. As a sensitive child, I was always sad when I went there. To face mortality at the age of nine, twelve or fifteen sucked.

While we ate our lunches in that cafeteria, it was always a great reminder of how lucky I was to have my health. Of course, five minutes after I left there, I snapped right back into the self-absorbed teenager that I was.

Mom never told me that she wanted me to appreciate my health. Maybe she truly thought the food was better in Children's Hospital cafeteria. Deep down I think she was teaching me a lesson that life is too precious to piss away. Whether you are four or ninety-seven, death can grab you anytime or anywhere.

When it came to the focus at home, I remember Dad getting me ready for school in the mornings or curling my hair on the day of school pictures. Mom kept long hours but because Dad had an outside sales job and then later owned his own metals company, he worked shorter hours. My father was paternal, caring and sweet, and my mother was a more serious person. My father liked to flow through life, while my mother was a doer, taking men's work roles in the 1970s and 80s. Her expertise did not come from doctoral level education but from hands-on experience. Mom loved learning. She educated herself in biotechnology, history, English literature and chemistry through the university's continuing education program.

What captured my mother's mind was history—her one true academic love. Once, for pure adventure and fun, she went on a Mississippi riverboat cruise with the famous Civil War historian and author, Shelby Foote. She had such a wonderful time that she still speaks of it today.

Mother loved to wear beautiful, amazing clothes. She would not spend a fortune on her wardrobe even though she looked like a million dollars. She was very practical about it because we didn't have a lot of money growing up. For a woman who loved to shop, she found consignment shops to browse through for her lovely wardrobe.

My dearest friend Cassie, who I've known since second grade, did a stint working in the lab for my mother while she was completing nursing school. Cassie described my mother as a well-dressed force of nature. When Mom walked through the sterile halls of the hospital, her 118 pounds of presence would take over the corridors. She was smart, pretty, well-spoken and armed with a reserved smile that told the person on the receiving end of one of her handshakes, "Mess with me and you'll be sorry."

My mother grew up on a farm and witnessed the death of animals throughout her childhood—a normal experience for life on the farm. Once, mom told me this sad story about her beloved dog Buck. He was a Boxer that my grandfather rescued as a puppy. Buck was an albino, all white, which meant that he would most certainly be deaf.

Somehow, Catherine's dad talked someone into giving him that albino puppy who turned out not to be deaf at all. He brought the dog home to my mom as a young girl, and she named him Buck. Buck was a great dog but he was not neutered; so Buck was not one to hang around the farm all day. The mischief Buck got into was never more than fighting a few male dogs and impregnating a few female dogs. That was normal dog behavior for Buck until he was six-years-old.

At age six, Buck killed a bunch of chickens on the next farm over. They knew it was Buck because he carried one of those dead chickens home as a gift to my mom. My grandfather was going to kill Buck right then, but my mother begged him not to. They tried to tie him up, but Buck had spent his whole life wandering the town. They even went as far as having him fixed, but nothing seemed to work. It was not even six months later when Buck got out again, went back to the same farm and killed the family cat this time.

That night when my grandfather finished working in the orange groves, he took Buck to the local vet and had him put to sleep. My grandfather knew that Buck meant the world to my mom, but he felt that being tied to a back porch would be no life for a dog that had spent his life running free. Buck could no longer be running wild as he always did. Despite the family's love for Buck, my grandfather decided that six years of a full life was better then six more years of living half a life being tied to a porch.

I think that mom's growing up on the farm honed certain strengths in her, but also hardness, not found in many women who wore five hundred dollar outfits to work each day. Her strength and a whole lot of smarts got her to where she was today

What I love most about my mom was something she said often:

> A woman's place in this world is wherever the
> hell she wants it to be.

You can be or do anything you put your mind to; just do it with as much grace and style as possible. That was my Mom.

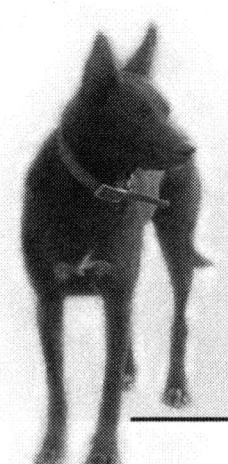

Chapter Three
Being Pregnant

If pregnancy were a book, they would cut the last two chapters.

~ Nora Ephron

Is Mine a Normal Pregnancy?

My pregnancy was routine, if you want to call looking six months pregnant during my first three months normal. I was *big*. My tummy wasn't the only part of my body that was growing; so were my buns, my thighs, my ankles and my breasts. You name the body part; it was swelling into ample size.

However, for the first time in my life I couldn't care less. I was 100% not embarrassed. I loved being pregnant and embraced the fact that two little ones were inside of me, needing nourishment. Long gone was the girl who lived on diet pills and two low-fat frozen dinners a day.

Wow, I was eating it all. As long as the food was good for

babies, it went into my mouth. I developed this huge fear about having tiny, little preemie twins. The only way I could combat this image in my head was to eat, eat and eat. I would eat my way to having big healthy twins.

No, I did not acquire this sage wisdom from a doctor, nurse or book. This was my own wacky idea. Even my mother kept telling me, "The bigger you get, the harder it will be to take off that weight." My crude response was, "I don't give a shit." I was going to have big, healthy babies, even if that meant that my butt would fill up my whole seat in the car by the time the pregnancy ran its course. My vanity of that once-size-six girl was gone! Here comes big mama!

Bed Rest? Not Me!

My other goal in this pregnancy was to avoid bed rest and to keep working. The bed rest part was out of my hands. I was forewarned from the books that I'd read that I had about a 50-50 chance that I would face bed rest.

I had the job aspect pretty well set. I was in sales and marketing of metals, specializing in exotic, hard-to-find metals. My boss also happened to be my father, Paul, the future grandfather of the little buns in my oven. I was able to prop my feet on my desk and eat all day if necessary without the boss discussing my new large look. Neither my father nor co-workers would frown on my running off to a two-hour obstetrics appointment. My fellow salesmen are my younger brother and my cousin. The rest of the staff, the office manager, and warehouse manager are like family to me. They had both worked for my father for over 18 years. Like me, they wanted to see the pregnancy go as smoothly as it could.

My life was full and blessed.

Barely Room Enough

Being one-third of the way through our pregnancy forced Robert and me to take a hard look at our housing reality. We had lived in a one-bedroom Palo Alto bungalow for a few years and had talked numerous times of remodeling. In the early years of this century, Silicon Valley was booming. People were making ridiculous amounts of money and enjoying life.

Robert and I had made many calls to contractors over time and found no willing jobbers. Contractors were building very expensive homes and people were paying cash for them. With our building budget of $100,000, we were not even a blip on any builder's radar. We couldn't get anyone who would add two bedrooms and a bathroom to our home.

Finally, we made arrangements with one design firm to remodel our home. When we gave them the deadlines, they said noncommittally, "We'll try our best." I didn't need that response with twins on the way. I really wanted to hear, "You got it. We guarantee it. Yes!"

Silly me, the eternal optimist! I turned my attention to finding a short-term rental. Keep in mind now that I am five months pregnant and we have five animals living with us. Would you rent to us? Neither would anyone else.

We only needed space for only four months but people would not consider a short-term rental in a very tight market as with our mortgage, remodeling payments and rental fees, the whole scenario was looking super-expensive.

I didn't want to invade my parent's privacy either. Their wonderful old farmhouse has plenty of space—for the two of them, their three dogs and nine cats. So we'd move in with our five animals? Didn't think so.

I said, "Well, they've got nine acres. We'll just rent a fifth wheel travel trailer and live on their nine acres." Then the funniest part of the pregnancy really unfolded.

One Big Happy Family

Robert and I stuck the biggest fifth wheel trailer available directly in front of my mother's house. She must have been mortified to wake up every morning and see this awful red, white, and blue trailer with advertising logos plastered on all sides. Although my parents' home is in the country, it is also adjacent to a park where people hike and ride horses. Those who travel the trails wave at mom and dad daily.

Despite the fact that the trailer had air conditioning, spending four hot summer months in a giant aluminum closet was an interesting scenario. I would spend time between work, the trailer and my parents' house cooling off because I seemed to constantly go into false labor and have contractions. I always seemed to be running back to the trailer to rest and prop my feet up.

One morning my ornery little terrier, Jeffrey, and I went outside. I could not see my own feet or the ground, so I paid attention when Jeffrey ran in front of my path and started barking madly. There was a baby rattlesnake right where I would step next. Jeffrey saved me!

One week later, I was floating and cooling off in my parents' pool. A bee stung me on the back, and my body slowly started to burn with fiery red bumps. I had an allergic reaction and couldn't reach my back or any other sensitive body part to scratch the hive-like welts. Thank goodness for prednisone.

Two weeks later, Jeffery wandered up to me with a swollen nose and face. The two marks on either side of his doggy face indicated bites from what I imagined to be a huge rattlesnake. I watched his little expression balloon up. What did I do?

I became hysterical and called my husband. Thinking I had gone into labor, he told me to calm down and get my mom on the phone so he could see if an ambulance was on its way. When I calmed down enough to explain that I was upset because Jeffery had stuck his nose in a snake hole and had been bitten by a rattlesnake, Robert pretty much lost it. Jeffery was not his favorite pet. He told me that if Jeffery caused me to go into premature labor he would personally shoot the dog himself.

Mom and I rushed Jeffrey to the vet. Robert met us there. They had one dose of antivenom left but we could not administer it there. The vet explained that we would have to buy the antivenom from them for $500 and then drive to the nearest animal *hospital* to have it administered so that Jeffery could be under observation for 24 hours. Robert did the math in his head and told the swollen faced Jeffery that he was not going to make it. I smacked my husband over the head—and paid for the antivenom. We all took off for the hospital.

At the animal hospital, a different veterinarian mixed the antivenom with adrenaline to prevent Jeffrey from going into anaphylactic shock. When she gave Jeffrey the injection, my husband was still upset with me, but Jeffrey would survive.

The female vet looked in my husband's eyes and said, "You know what? I've seen many people come in here, and they're much more hysterical with their pets because they can't explain to them what's going on. Pets don't understand. And the same thing may happen with a baby. At least with children, you can explain it a little better."

She was a mother and told my husband where to stick it. Jeffrey turned out to be all right after several days. I am not sure my husband returned to normal though.

Growing Larger as Time Grows Short

I was *so* pregnant in September 2001. The babies were due in a month. I am 5' 7" in height and was pushing 200 pounds with a very rounded abdomen. Thank heavens our big bed accommodated me with my two dogs, three cats and Robert.

However, I couldn't fit in the tiny trailer's bathroom anymore, meaning I had to back in to sit on the john. And forget about the shower. It was so small and I was so big that I could only wash half of me at a time. Evidently, this was fairly comical to watch but I just found it be cold. I wanted to be back in my own home.

Remember the design firm that said they would "try" to be finished by September. Well, they completed the remodeling in the nick of time! We moved out of the trailer and into our newly remodeled home two weeks before our due date of October 31st.

However, one more major event rocked our world before we moved from my parents' property.

Chapter Four

Then the World Shuddered

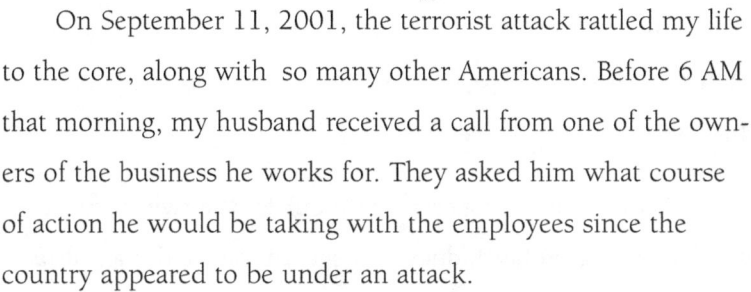

You can be sure that the American spirit will prevail over this tragedy.

~ Colin Powell

On September 11, 2001, the terrorist attack rattled my life to the core, along with so many other Americans. Before 6 AM that morning, my husband received a call from one of the owners of the business he works for. They asked him what course of action he would be taking with the employees since the country appeared to be under an attack.

Robert and I turned on the one television station that we could get out in the country. I witnessed a sight that will stay in my mind until the day I die. One of the World Trade Center buildings was burning from a plane that recently flew into it. Then suddenly—slam! Another airplane flies directly into the other World Trade building.

We quickly got dressed and ran to my parents' home to see on their big TV screen these unreal events unfold like a horrific dream. My mother, Robert and I sat mesmerized; unable to understand how or why someone would kill so many innocent people.

Then the unthinkable happened. The Twin Towers fell to the ground. First one crumbled, and then the next. I was frozen in shock, unable to cry. So many people trapped in and under the building.

I couldn't stand it any longer. Suddenly, in the middle of all the madness, I stood up and said, "Mom, Robert, I just can't sit here like this. I am going for my ultrasound appointment."

"Jenn, you will not leave this house under any circumstances. For God's sake Jenn, we are under attack!" Robert pleaded.

We were having concerns with our female twin because she had a spot on her kidney and every time we did an ultrasound it looked like she had a cleft pallet. I needed to be prepared for that in case a surgeon had to be scheduled so close to the delivery time. Yet, we could never get a good look at her face; usually if there's fluid on the kidney it can mean hand deformities or facial deformities. So I needed to keep this appointment and stay focused on the babies.

Robert remained adamant, "Well, you can't leave. I have to go to work so you just reschedule your appointment."

"Absolutely not. I can't just stop my life right now because of this. I have to take control of my own situation."

"This is crazy. You can't go."

What was crazy to me was arguing about the babies' safety. I got my purse and walked out. The children were most important for me. I was in shock at that point anyway, but stable enough to know my priorities.

Empty Spaces

When I arrived for my appointment at the doctor's office, the waiting room was silent and empty. The two exceptions were the woman who looked like she could go into labor at any time and the receptionist at the front desk.

As I went into the ultrasound room, I noticed the technician who was always so happy and full of kind words looked pale. She was silent while she started the ultrasound procedures. Tears rolled down her cheeks in a steady flow.

"It is an awful day, isn't it?" I said, inviting her to open up a little.

"Yes." So sadly she turned to me. "Well, you know what?

Your kids look great. I see this spot still on here but they are absolutely perfect. This is something that, you know, that is making today okay."

Being a mother, I had put everything else on hold in the world to consider my children first. Yet, the real world was out there seemingly lying in wait.

After the appointment I sat in the parking lot listening to National Public Radio. For the next hour, I could finally let the well of tears run its course. Other mothers like me surely wept for all the children who lost their mommies and daddies; for all the suffering that friends must feel and the uncertainty this country faced. My babies heard my whispers: *What kind of world are you coming into? Are you crying with me? Thank you for being my babies.*

I could feel the collective souls of everyone in America shuddering.

In the following hours and days, my mother and dad, Robert and I felt cut off in the country. We read the news when we had a chance at work or we would listen to the radio in the car.

That week was our last in the trailer at the farm. Our newly renovated home beckoned us to prepare for the twins' arrival. Our time in the pastoral scenery on my parents' nine acres, away from our cosmopolitan neighborhood, was one of the most peaceful times of my life. The terrorist attack shattered that serenity and brought up a mom's fears about what kind of world I was bringing children into.

Chapter Five

Welcome New Souls!

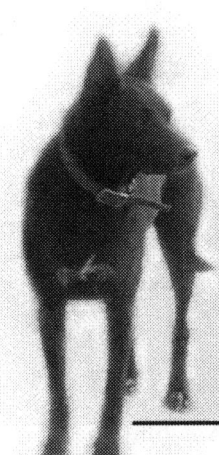

I'm not interested in being Wonder Woman in the delivery room. Give me drugs.   ~ Madonna

Help!

Eager to return home, I was ready to tackle the nursery and get the beds, strollers, highchairs and all baby paraphernalia assembled. We had to prepare two of everything! However, I couldn't bend or reach, and my range of vision was limited to what was in front of my nose. Besides that, I was to stay seated with my feet propped up.

What's a mom to do? I called my five best girlfriends and asked for help. All of them came over to put together cribs and strollers and more. I am so grateful for their support.

Unfortunately, as time went on, some of the pieces they

assembled started to fall apart. I was pushing the kids in the stroller after they were born and one of the wheels fell off. I was able to get it back on without tipping the kids out of their seats, but it was not easy. A bookshelf also broke. Once it was turned on, most the pieces on the mobile kept falling off. Each drawer in the dresser was off its tracks and would not open or close properly. All four of the drawers were cockeyed in different directions. The toy box they built that was supposed to stay propped open (when opened all the way) would only stay open on one side. This would cause the side that was assembled incorrectly to quickly fall back onto to toy box. Watching the toy box lid slam back into the box gave me horrible visions of one of the twins' heads getting smashed. Thank goodness they didn't have time to build the cribs!

I could not ask for a better group of girlfriends; I love each of them to death. But none of them should think about getting into carpentry as a line of work.

Arrival

Thirty-six weeks, three days plus sixteen hours of labor later, my quest to have children ended happily with the birth of a beautiful boy and girl. My son weighed in at 6 lbs 7 oz, and my daughter was 6 lbs. Robert and I felt such joy to have these healthy babies.

The twins went off to the hospital nursery that first night so I could get some rest and Robert could go home. Realty kicked in, however, the next night when I kept them with me. I fed them by myself for the first time.

I mumbled through tired tears, "How am I going to do this?" I spent a lot of time crying that night. More than anything else, I was scared to death that these two tiny bundles both needed me at the same time.

I did manage to get them fed and survived the second night. I felt like the Great Mommy Goddess should give me a gold star, such was the simple, yet wonderful feeling of accomplishing the first tasks of motherhood.

The next day when my husband and family showed up with smiles and support, I realized that we were going to be just fine.

Chapter Six

Complications

I trust that everything happens for a reason, even when we're not wise enough to see it. ~ Oprah Winfrey

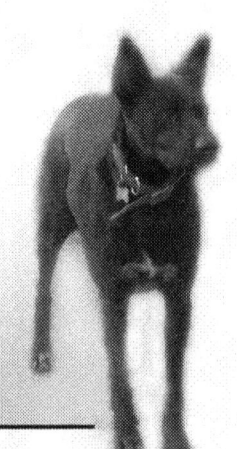

Welcome Home

When I started writing this book, other moms asked me what twin babies are really like. How did I manage? Who helped? How did I handle schedules for two babies? When I try to remember, I'm amazed that the first two years of their lives seems like the blur of a movie on fast-forward. To capture specific frames is difficult because of the traumatic events that happened within my family.

In the beginning, life with the kids went on normally. Robert took that first week off after they were born and that was it.

Robert is the vice-president of an 80-person environmental

services company that had grown from 15 employees when he started. He wears a lot of the hats in his position and is at one of their three main California offices every single weekday. Maybe he takes two weeks off throughout the year.

Robert derives much happiness from succeeding in work and always seems to have high energy. He can give 110% throughout his whole day at work and still have energy and enthusiasm for his children when he gets home. He loves being a dad.

Robert and I developed an understanding that he would work and I would be the children's main caregiver, even when I went back to work as my son and daughter grew older. So in those early years, Monday through Fridays were my days and Robert helped on the weekends.

Illness Strikes in Threes

Right after the children were born, my mom took off eight weeks from work. Four weeks would be spent at our house to help care for the twins, and then she would have a minor knee operation with four more weeks to recover at home.

My son was very ill with gastric reflux, which is like heartburn in an immature digestive system. He was regurgitating everything. We had to take him back to the hospital for a night of observation. The solution to his problem was an over-the-counter antacid and an hourly feeding schedule. He was to be given one ounce of formula or breast milk every hour for three weeks. I started my routine of setting the alarm clock to go off every hour, day and night for three weeks. My mom helped with Anna during the day and Robert helped some at night but it was pretty much all me. I can hardly remember this period now.

I was exhausted and hardly producing any milk. The guilt was killing me. I felt like I was harming my babies by depriving them of the best possible start they could have. Doctors, nurses, family and friends pressured me. "Just breastfeed," they would say. Their advice grew so out of control that I was amazed at how much people felt that this was their business. Then one day, my brother looked at me and said, "You're yellow and gray." I did feel horrible and needed to go to the hospital. I was jaundiced, had high blood pressure, and felt excruciating abdominal pain.

I had to laugh as I described the pain to the doctors as "horrible as labor." Then I threw up. Through an ultrasound, they found that my gall bladder was obstructed, and I needed surgery immediately to have it removed. Ouch. I finally understood why I was feeling so crummy and exhausted. I was very sick.

A week later, my husband took me to the surgicenter while

my mom and dad took care of the kids. The surgery went fine although the outpatient procedure turned into an overnight visit so they could keep an eye on me. My first night in bed alone in weeks! (Incidentally my husband still counts this as a night "away" as if I was at some Napa Valley spa with friends.)

Shortly after my surgery, my son recovered from his reflux. With my surgery out of the way and my baby boy on the mend, we looked forward to some calmer days ahead. Mom's routine knee surgery was next on the agenda.

Chapter Seven

Losing Mom

Time is the only comforter for the loss of a mother. ~ Jane Welsh Carlyle

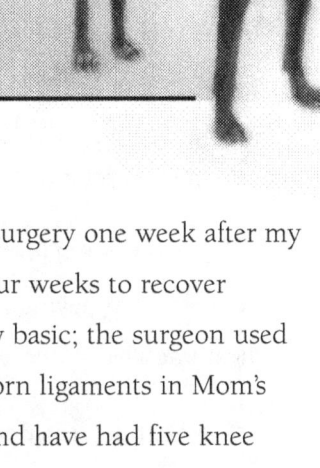

Mom had her arthroscopic knee surgery one week after my gall bladder surgery, still giving her four weeks to recover before returning to work. It was pretty basic; the surgeon used a small camera to see and repair the torn ligaments in Mom's knee. I inherited her crummy knees and have had five knee surgeries myself. I was more of an extreme athlete so I kept beating them down. Because of our experiences, none of us were worried about Mom's surgery.

Within the first twenty-four hours of her surgery, there were no complications. By the second day, Mom was at home and lying in bed. Her leg was propped up and had swollen from the surgery.

While my father was getting ready to go to work, Mom said goodbye to the friend she had been speaking on the phone with, stood up and slowly walked into her bathroom where she had trouble breathing and collapsed to the floor.

In some moment of lucidity, Mom yelled for Dad who was just walking inside the house after being out with the horses. Mom could barely talk. I think at that point the blood clot had gone into her lung causing shortness of breath. When Dad came in, Mom managed to say she was having a heart attack.

Dad called 911. The emergency medical technicians arrived and mom must have realized at that point that she was not having a heart attack.

She told the EMTs, "You know what? I had knee surgery. I threw a clot. I'm having a pulmonary aneurysm." Would Mom's medical knowledge and experience save her life?

"We can't get a strong pulse on you. We think you're having a heart attack."

"No, that's not it." Mom insisted. "This is what's going on with me right now and you need to get clot-busters."

The EMTs rushed Mom into the ambulance and called ahead to the closest hospital. They explained to her, "We have to take you there. We're losing your pulse." When she tried to protest to be taken to the hospital where she worked, the EMTs responded, "That one is farther away and you're not going to make it."

Rushing

Kate, a woman who worked with Mom and was renting the cottage on my parent's ranch, called us at our house. She reached my mother-in-law and father-in-law who had been staying with us for the past week, visiting with the twins. I was taking a shower when my husband came down and said, "Kate called and your mother has either had a heart attack or a pulmonary embolism." As I ran upstairs, rushing to get out the door, my mother-in-law said, "Well, let's hope it's not a heart attack."

My response was "No, let's hope that's it's not a pulmonary embolism because she'll be dead by the time we get there if it is."

While Robert and I raced to the hospital, I called my eighty-four-year-old grandmother, Mom's mother, in Idaho. My grandmother is mentally present, strong, and she's got a deep faith in the Catholic Church and in God. Sometimes I think people of such deep faith weather adverse events in a better way than most.

"Well, you know what?" Grandmother said, "You call me and you tell me what's going on because I need to know. I'm going to sit here and pray for her. Just let me know and when you get a chance, you have to call me." Grandmother took it well. She wasn't too upset.

When Robert and I arrived at the hospital, my father announced, "Nobody call Grandma." I'm like, "Oh, great." I didn't say anything, not a word, because I knew Grandma could handle it. She is such a strong woman like my mother.

Fearful of the Worst

By the time Mom had arrived at the emergency room, she was almost gone. The doctor pulled her back in and prepared to intubate her. She opened her eyes. The doctor said to her, "So you think you're having a pulmonary embolism? So do I."

Mom looked at the doctor and replied, "No shit. Of course that's what I'm having."

"Okay, we're putting the medicine in right now" he told her and my Mom's eyes closed.

Then Mom flat-lined and died right there on the table in the emergency room. The doctors began working on her furiously shocking her body and giving her adrenaline and oxygen.

We were unaware of all this as we waited in the emergency room lobby, but as the minutes passed, we became desperate for information. Any information. Finally, we spied the doctor down the hall looking directly at us. He invited us into a private room to speak with him. I thought he was merely being polite. It didn't dawn on me that this was the hospital protocol for families of the dying.

The doctor followed behind us and closed the door. "Well, it doesn't look good," he said.

"You know, what do you mean it doesn't look good? How can… she's perfectly healthy." I stuttered through my thoughts aloud. "This is the woman who discovered yoga ten years ago and practices it every other day. Mom was physically strong from riding horses, carrying bales of hay, walking. She had this farm and worked…"

He broke in, "We've been working on her for 30 minutes. She's still down. We're keeping her heart beating artificially right now."

After a pregnant pause, he continued, "We have her blood so thinned out that, you know, we're hoping we busted the clot, but we don't know. In fact, I need to go back down there, because she's still technically not dead, but I'm sure she's not going to make it." The doctor left.

I could only scream, grab my brother's and my husband's hand and sit down. In that particular moment, the person I thought of was not my mother, but my dad. I felt so horrible that he might be all alone. My brother and I were there with our spouses. Dad stood alone and silent. Was he reflecting on the early years? He and Mom had been together since they were twenty years old.

Regaining some composure, I stood up, looked at my dad and asked, "What can I get you? What do you need?"

"Some aspirin, please."

I walked over to the pharmacy and got Dad his aspirin. The doctor was in the room again when I returned.

Can It Get Worse?

The doctor spoke with us quietly and respectfully: "Well, we have more bad news. We have her heart working again, but now she's gone into DIC. She's bleeding out."

DIC stands for disseminated intravascular coagulopathy, an unfortunate side effect of using clot-busters. Doctors had thinned her blood out so much that she was now bleeding onto the brain and everywhere else. They cut her clothes off because they were so soaked in blood.

So my Dad told me to call her boss, who was the head of cardiac surgery at University Medical Center. Because it was Sunday morning, I thought I would not be able to reach him. I walked outside and used my cell phone to call his hospital and explain the situation: "My mother works for Dr. Ted Moss and you need to connect me to him. I know he's off today. He's at home. But, you know, I have to talk to him." And they did track him down.

Ted was kind enough to call me back. I explained the situation to him and I said, "This is what happened and now she is in DIC and she is bleeding."

"No, that's impossible."

"Yes, that's what the doctor said." At that point, Ted thought that they would probably give her 1 chance in 1,000 of surviving.

I returned to the private room to join the others. Another hour passed. The doctor returned and told us that they had finally stabilized Mom and were moving her to ICU. However, the damage had been done. She had been down a total of 42 minutes. Her brain was not working.

The Waiting Game

I called Mom's friend, Sue, who had worked with her for 20 years at University Hospital as well as Caitlin and Val. These three nurses, who ran the transplant department, came over immediately. Sue held together well, but her friend, Caitlin, really didn't. They went into ICU to see Mom and were pretty torn up about her.

When they returned they said, "You know, you need to see your mother.

"I can't go see her." I had been there five hours at that point. I was strained to the max.

"She looks really bad, but you have to because, you know, she can probably hear you. You need to say goodbye to her because she's not going to live."

I heeded their words. They were right, but to say goodbye to your mother…? I was not prepared for this. No one is prepared for this. I went in. She was so blown up with medication that her fingers were ten times the size of a regular finger. Her fingers were oozing blood out the ends. Her eyes, nose and her ears were bloated; she was oozing blood and medicine out of all her orifices. It was a horrific sight.

The thought that this would be the last memory of my mother seemed incomprehensible to me. I was so tired. I tried to talk to her. Then I just had to leave.

That night, the neurologist reiterated to us that she had no brainwaves; she had been down way too long. There is no way she was going to come back. The doctor suggested that we give Mom a few days before we make any bigger decisions about her life support or organ donations.

I sent my husband back home to rejoin his parents and take care of the twins. My brother and I went back to my parents' house to spend the night with Dad. I couldn't go into their bedroom because that was the last place she was before she collapsed. Her bathrobe was still in her bed.

Dad slept on the couch. I slept in the other bedroom and my brother slept in their room. Yet, no one slept that night.

In the morning, Dad reminded us that Mom had requested that if she was in a vegetative state, we were to pull the plug and let her die and donate her organs.

Dad fed the horses and we returned to the hospital. Mom was still alive. Her condition was unchanged, but now we had another neurologists' opinion about her condition. Mom's boss had arrived at 6AM that morning to examine her and had also determined that she was probably not coming back.

I called my grandmother again to keep her in the loop. "Grandma, mom is probably not going to live, and I'm not supposed to tell you that, so just talk to me. Dad didn't want to upset you, so please don't talk to anyone else about it." My father would have been furious at me because he didn't want grandmother to be upset; yet I knew she had the stamina.

The next day mom's condition was unchanged. She was still on the ventilator and registered as brain-dead. She was too unstable to move to University Hospital, which is where Mom would want to be. We had to keep her in the ICU for a few more days.

Then we transferred Mom to University Hospital's ICU where she could be in the care of those with whom she worked. The staff promised to take care of everything. The first thing her boss did was to put her in a medically induced coma. He explained, "What we need to do is put her in a really deep sleep. She needs to rest. Her brain has all this blood on it along with the other problems. She needs to sleep. If she comes out of this, then she'll come out. Otherwise, you know that's it."

The other consulting neurologists basically said, "She's not going to wake up. She is brain-dead. You can give it a little more time, but this is the reality of the situation. When we take the ventilator out, she's going to die."

My father said to one German neurologist, "You know she's on a lot of medication and she is very affected by it. I really think she might wake up."

She replied, "You know what? I think she might, too. I don't know what her mind is going to be like, but I too think she might come out of it." She was the only one who had an intuitive sense about it, as my father had. Everybody else said,

"No way."

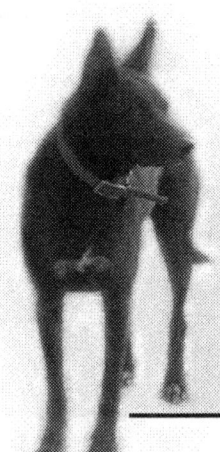

Chapter Eight

Dad

Blessed indeed is the man who hears many gentle voices call him father!

~ Lydia M. Child

While Mom was in a coma, there were days that we thought would be her last because her brain consistently showed no activity. A daughter experiences so much grief in the anticipation of her mother's death. Truly the waiting was the most difficult part of this journey.

I was heartbroken to think that my children might never know the grandmother who loved them so dearly. I hired a nanny to stay with the children during the day so I could be by my mom's bedside. During this sad time, my only bright moments came when I returned home every couple of hours to see my babies. The stress took its toll and I became rundown and tired. I attributed it to the overload of taking care of the twins, dealing with my mother's illness and worrying about my Dad.

The only thought more heartbreaking to me than losing my young, healthy, amazing Mom was the thought of my dad losing his wife of thirty-three years. They had a great marriage—the real deal. They were two of the most different people in the world, yet they worked seamlessly as a team. Unlike my powerful, fun, yet no nonsense mother, my father had a whole different approach on how he lived his life. My father is a generous man who is filled with wonderful stories that illustrate kindness and humor.

Immigrants

These are the stories my father told me as a child; these stories made my father seem the forever-dreamer of a better tomorrow. My father's dad, Louis Philip (a.k.a. Lou) was born in the United States in 1903. His family of Russian Jews immigrated to the United States in 1890 to escape the pogrom massacres in Russia. My grandfather's family name was Gruhin, which was changed to Greene somewhere in the Ellis Island registration procedures.

My grandfather's first wife taught at a school of dance. What truthfully happened between them, we'll never know, but some family members believe that she didn't want children.

One day, grandfather went to visit his brother at the hospital pharmacy. There grandfather met Mary who was working as a nurse's aid at the hospital. Mary was a fresh-faced twenty-one-year-old just a few years off the boat from Ireland. Mary Catherine McDermott emigrated from Ireland at age 17 in 1929 and was also escaping persecution. My grandmother's family lived near Northern Ireland and saw friends and family members killed by British soldiers because of The Troubles in Ireland between the English Protestants and the Irish Catholics.

As the story goes, Lou fell madly in love with Mary when he first set eyes on her. Then, they went through hell and back to make the love they had for one anther work. People of different faiths did not marry. Both Lou and Mary felt the persecutions of being Jewish and Irish Catholic and the disfavor of their families for their spousal choices.

My grandmother was ten years younger than my grandfather when they married in the mid-1930s. As a young woman fresh from Ireland, she carried much guilt about marrying a divorced non-Catholic and was concerned about properly raising her children in the Church. My grandfather did not convert to Catholicism at the time of their marriage. Their first son was born in 1936.

The story goes that Grandmother had a nervous breakdown by the time of their second child's arrival. As a result grandfather converted and became a super-Catholic, perhaps in the extreme. My father's parents built a chapel in the backyard at their house in Southern California. Every night, the family had to go to the chapel and say the rosary together.

As a boy, my father loved Flash Gordon. He was often furious when the evening Rosary took precedence over the TV show, but my grandfather would not let him skip this ritual.

My grandfather would recite the rosary as he drove down the Los Angeles highways of those days. Super-Catholic also meant that the words of the Bible were influential in the lives of their eight children.

At the same time, my grandparents were incredibly generous people who took care of their own. If any of their friends, family or people they met were in trouble or needed help, they would take care of them. They would send money back to Ireland. They donated money to build tennis courts for their local girls' Catholic school.

My grandfather was a forward thinking man who made his money through a variety of businesses. He had a caster business in east or central Los Angeles. He hired Latinos or African Americans from within the community at a time when other businesses would only hire Caucasian workers. My grandfather firmly believed that one didn't judge people by the color of their skin or their religion. He had grown up in a time when it was not unusual to see in windows of many businesses, "No shirts, no shoes, no Jews." My grandparents were devoted to the Catholic Church, which held its followers to live by prescribed standards—they truly lived by Christian principles.

Grandfather owned another business called the Store of Surprises, where they bought clothes from the department stores and sold them like a high-end thrift store. Lou was truly a one of a kind.

When I went to Ireland at the age of 17, the people of the small little town where my grandmother was from still remembered both of them. It had been many years since Lou had been back to Manorhamilton, but the family and the people of the town described him so clearly, it was as if he had been there yesterday. I would get introduced as "Mary McDermott's granddaughter from California." Everyone would say, "Ah, Mary, what a lovely woman, and that husband of hers, Lou, what a good man he was, indeed." And the most wonderful thing that everyone would also say is that he was a generous man with such a big heart.

I am sure that before they had come to know Lou, they may have been a bit taken back. He was probably the first New Yorker to have visited the small rural town when my grandmother took him back there in the late 1930's. Very unlike the Irish farmers at the time, he would talk to anyone and everyone. Everything he did was at a very fast pace. No one could keep up with the man, the way he walked and talked. I can just envision him walking up to some farmer, tired at the end of his long day working out at the bogs, or sitting down to have a pint next to a local at the village pub, and announcing without any hesitation "Hi, I am Lou Greene from New York City. It's nice to meet you." He probably could have told them he was from Mars—Mars being no more foreign at that time than New York to the folks of Manorhamilton. No matter, over time he won them over.

My grandfather died when I was a toddler. I've come to know my grandfather through my grandmother. When I was seven years old, I asked grandmother, "Why didn't you ever get remarried?"

She looked shocked, but she responded, "I am married to your grandfather."

"Well he's been gone a long time."

She stared at me a little longer, and then replied in a quiet voice, "I married the man I loved, and, what more could a person want? I am so lucky to have had that. Of course I would never remarry." Even at that age, I knew I had offended her somehow, but she responded to me graciously.

Later in her life I helped Grandmother. I spoke with her on the telephone several times a day. I would make her appointments for the dentist or doctor for her and arranged her transportation.

Grandmother didn't have much money anymore. To thank me, she would give me the romantic letters that grandfather sent her. She would share wonderful stories. I loved to read these wonderful romantic love letters her wrote her. It would make me feel closer to a man whom I would never know.

My grandmother occasionally drank with the indulgence of her Irish background. The first time I ever got drunk was with my grandmother. When I was 11 years old, she needed an escort to go to a wedding back in New Jersey for one of my dad's cousins. So I escorted her to this huge Irish Catholic wedding where she let me drink. She said, "It's okay. Have the time of your life. Whatever…"

My parents were mortified when they saw the family pictures, and their young daughter was grinning with a Margarita in her hand. The funny thing about that, Grandmother never let me drink again.

Best of Both Parents

During his senior year of high school, some college scouts came to see my dad play football and run track. The scouts were enthusiastic about him until his grade point average came up. School academics were not Dad's forte, but sports were. He is a smart, well-read guy, but did not click with the formal education that the nuns provided.

After high school, Dad bounced around from junior college to junior college. He would play football and run track, then move on to a different junior college. He did all this while still working for at Grandfather's business.

After a few years of jumping around from team to team (rather than school to school), my mom entered the picture. Four months later they were married. I arrived the following year!

My father's Catholic upbringing soured him on the dogma of God and heaven. He would say: "Simply you live, simply you die, and that's it, nothing more."

In his heart, day in and day out, Dad is truly a blessed person. He has values that so many of us are missing, like an uncontested drive of good intentions toward all living creatures.

In addition to his family, the great loves of my father's life have been animals—mostly dogs. I can't remember a time in my life when our house not was filled with dogs, cats, hamsters and snakes.

Every night, dad would take his dogs out for walks around the neighborhood that might last an hour or longer. He always told me that it was the dogs' time. This meant that no bush went un-sniffed and no spot unmarked. He never pulled them along, or made them rush through the walk. He just let them set the pace.

For the last 25 years, when people dump cats next to his business in Mountain View, California, he adopts them and insures that they are neutered or spayed. This love for cats and dogs goes back to his childhood when he brought home stray pets. He installed a cat door at work and provides food for them. This can be a little shocking for new customers. Some days, there are literally more cats wandering around the office than employees. Since many of them were born feral, most would struggle to place in a traditional cat show. But we love them all very much and give them names like Meeky, Meesee, Orange Fluff-Bucket, Jesse James, Tabby Cat, Lefty, Scrappy, Scruffy and Mongo. One of my favorites was so disheveled she looked like an extra from Pet Cemetery. Since she was an older cat, we named her Gray Momma. She lived to be about 20.

Dad also believes in supporting a shelter for battered women and children, and insuring that during the non-school years, the children in the shelter are fed. My father has a generous and kind heart for numerous other causes.

Growing Up with Dad

I feel that Dad and I have a strong heart connection. Even though as a child or teen, I didn't understand his motives, as an adult, I truly appreciate that he cared as he did.

For example, when I was in middle school and high school, I'd sneak out to go to parties. Some parents let their kids go; my dad said, "No, absolutely you can't go." So, when my parents went to bed, I would sneak out the window.

Dad would drive around at night until he found me. He would always find the party, and that's what got me. I don't know how he found me. He'd come into the party and everyone would say, "Oh, Jenny, your dad's here." I was mortified. Every single time he would come out and find me, and he was the only parent that did that.

Another event that reminds me of Dad's values was a time we were walking Malcolm, one of our dogs. At fourteen, I tried my best line, "Dad this party tonight—I have to go. I'm not going to drink or smoke. I promise you. This is the best party. I can't miss it. Everyone's going."

Dad says, "You know, you're always going to think you're missing the best party, but you never slow down and you never appreciate the little things like walking the dog right now. This is great."

I looked at him blankly. "You know, Dad, I'm not talking about walking the dog. I'm talking about a party," I said.

"No, I'm talking about you needing to slow down and starting to appreciate the little things in life because you're not doing it right now."

That stuck with me forever because Dad was so serious when he told me what he honestly believed. It took me a long time to know what he was talking about, but it did finally sink in.

Room to Grow Up

I had a really hard time in school when I was growing up because of a learning disability. I am extremely dyslexic. I went to boarding schools and private schools. Finally, I dropped out of school when I was seventeen and moved to Europe.

Now that I have children, I am not sure I would let my kids do something like that. However, my parents may have determined that I needed to find myself. Due in large part to my learning disability, I had become fiercely independent at the age of 17. Traveling around Europe allowed me to experience cultures and life in a different venue. I needed that exposure.

I realized on that trip that I needed to get a college education because I had walked away from high school with almost no formal education. I did some research and found Landmark College in Vermont, the only college for dyslexics in the world. I was ecstatic. My parents agreed to pay for tuition so I applied and was accepted.

Landmark was life-changing experience for me. The first

time I called my dad, I was crying. I said, "For the first time in my life I'm actually learning. I can do this. I can actually do school work. I can't thank you enough."

Dad started crying and handed the phone to my mother because he couldn't talk. That was the only time that's ever happened where he couldn't talk to me.

In this two-year college, I took the basic study skills program and learned how to learn. I also took some accredited programs and then transferred to a four-year college, where I eventually earned a bachelor's degree in Humanities.

After that, I went to work for my father, only planning to stay for a year while I acquired my teaching certificate. Well, 12 years later, I am still there. It is a warm and wonderful place to work.

As a teenager, I found my Dad's stories about life somewhat dull. I did not understand the value of what he was trying to tell me until I became an adult. For example, the simplicity of a nice dinner with your family or a quiet walk with your dog is what can make a day perfect. Appreciating the little things in your life can truly fill you with happiness.

His values and kindness extend to everyone he encounters everyday. He is even nice to telemarketers who call him at work or at home. At work, I still ask why he doesn't just hang up on pushy stockbrokers or sales calls. He replies, "They are just trying to do their job. Why would I hang up on them? That would be rude."

You know, he's right. Taking an extra few moments out of your day to simply say, "No, thank you, have a nice day." would not kill any of us.

The biggest lesson I learned from Dad is to try and find enjoyment and laughter everywhere I can.

Chapter Nine

And Then Came Arthur

I think dogs are the most amazing creatures; they give unconditional love. For me they are the role-model for being alive. ~ Gilda Radner

---

The day after we spoke to the German neurologist, Dad arrived at the hospital and reported that he had found a dog. He casually mentioned to me, "Oh I found this dog, and it is in really bad shape. He's basically feral. I'm going to take him to the shelter."

When he said he was taking the dog to the shelter, I felt a sensation like a rubber band snapping against my chest. My mouth flew open. "Well you can't do that, you know. They're just going to put him down."

My father loves dogs, but he was so burden with everything going on right then, he couldn't think about taking on a dog.

"What do you think I'm going to do?" he asked pointedly. "I've got to take care of the property. I've got to take care of my business, and most importantly, I've got to take care of your mother."

"Dad, you can't. They'll just put down an unsocialized dog like him. This dog came to you for a reason. You saved his life for a reason Dad! Maybe God sent you this dog."

Now I had done it. Not only did I use guilt to try to make this man, whose life was completely upside down, keep a dog, I used the dreaded three-letter word: G-O-D!

"What is wrong with you Jennifer? Your mother could die at any second. I am trying to run my company and maintain a farm. You are telling *me*, God, a huge load of BS created to keep order in society, would send me a half-dead feral dog?"

Dad wasn't too happy with me. He left Mom's room, letting me know in no uncertain terms that he was sure I had lost my mind.

I don't think I've ever seen my Dad look at me in such a pissed-off way before that day. He has been a devout atheist his whole adult life and made no bones about the nonexistence of God. According to Dad, when you die, you go in the ground. There has never been any proof of God's existence. Because he was preached to so hard by his parents, religion, and especially

Catholicism, was just such a bunch of hypocrisy.

During this time of my mother's illness, people were continually coming up to me and saying, "I'm praying for your mother." I had the weirdest sensations; I could feel this energy of people praying for her. Was I just feeling incredible grief? Was I seeking comfort? Or did I really feel the energetic buzz of others supporting my Mom through prayer? When people said that they were praying for my mother, I felt a warm glow envelope me, almost hug me. This wonderful feeling brought me overwhelming calmness and a positive healing feeling.

At the moment of our dog conversation, I felt like the dog could help save my father in some way, because my father couldn't save my mother. I felt Dad needed that hope more than anything because he felt so hopeless. With everything around him falling apart, here came this half-dead dog that Dad could save.

After we had the big argument at the hospital, he left and never mentioned our conversation again. He was really mad at me.

However, the next day, when Dad arrived at the hospital, he said, "Well, Arthur and I…" I interrupted him and asked, "Who is Arthur?"

"Well, the dog" he said. Dad had named the dog Arthur. I

was glad because that meant he wasn't getting rid of him now. He named him. That's it. I knew that Arthur was here to stay.

Arthur looked half-starved. Someone had probably dumped him in the open space preserve next to my parents place. He's a McNabb mix—a kind of herding dog. Who knows what he's mixed with, but he's definitely a McNabb. Arthur had thirty-two ticks on him and was not well socialized, but he wasn't mean.

Because my father had seven cats, there was concern of bringing an unsocialized dog onto the property. But my dad could not just ignore him because he was in such bad shape. Dad gave him food and water and kept him in the barn next to the horses that night because he had no idea how he would react to his older dogs, Hobbes and Magen, or the seven cats.

Dad moved Arthur into the main house a few nights later. He never fought with my Dad's older dog, Hobbs. Arthur also got along with the cats, blending in with the rest of the family, and found his place on the farm.

Hobbs died not too long after Arthur's arrival. Even though Dad loves all of his dogs, he loved Hobbs the most, and having Arthur made the transition a little bit easier.

Arthur needed to keep order on the farm. If the other dogs were being too loud or out of line, like when I brought my dogs down, Arthur kept them in line. He didn't hurt them; he barked and held them down with his paw. When they got quiet, he got back on his porch and returned to keeping his lookout.

Arthur could be cranky too. Two years after he arrived, my Dad got another McNabb puppy and she just drives Arthur crazy. Sometimes he just grumps around.

I know Arthur was dumped there, but I believe there was for a reason he showed up shortly after Mom had her stroke. My dad needed something. He needed something to give him hope. I don't know if there is or isn't a God. What I do know is that Arthur blended into the family as if he were always meant to be there. Arthur stepped up as the alpha dog of the house and the new watchdog of the farm. Arthur gave my dad someone to go home to after all the long days at the hospital.

Dad deserved this gift. He simply goes through his life, day in and day out, touching all those around him by being a good person. No hype about it. He acts the way he does because of goodness inside him that so many people in this world lack. This is why God gave him a dog. Dogs are creatures so good, loyal and trustworthy—just like my father. That's why God sent Arthur.

Chapter Ten

Where There's a Will, There's a Way

A woman is like a tea bag. You never know how strong she is until she gets in hot water.

~ Eleanor Roosevelt

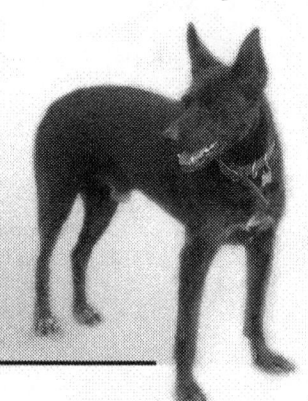

Seeing mom in a coma, helpless in a hospital bed, left all of us feeling at a loss for what to do except to rise each morning and let mom know we were still with her.

We believed she could hear us, so we talked to her as though she could. Privately we asked ourselves why she hadn't died; and if she did continue to live, by some blessing, what would be her future quality of life. If it were poor, how would my father care for her, his business and the farm?

So many questions remained unanswered. What we were left with was faith in her strong spirit and tenacity. I imagined the young horsewoman who rode through the fragrant orange groves, exhilarated by her love of land and horses.

The last time I had been in Mom's childhood home was twenty years ago when Mom's father became ill with cancer.

My mother, brother and I would drive the hour or so to my grandparent's orange grove to water and take care of the property. When we arrived, my brother and I could not wait to take off our shoes and run around in the deep, thick muddy irrigation ruts that ran between the orange trees. I don't know how many acres were there, but they stretched as far as a child's eye could see.

So Mom would work and my brother and I would swing from the old orange trees, now covered in warm soft mud from the water irrigation, with the hot Southern California sun beating down on us. I love my grandparents old farmhouse, to me, it was the perfect place for a child to spend there summers.

Not much later, my grandfather died and the orange groves and the old house were sold. I was too young to remember if mom was sad to let go of such an amazing place. I know my mom's family put their blood and sweat into the groves with little payback. Selling the land and her home must have been heartbreaking for her.

Or maybe she was ready to move on to the next phase of her life. In the few short weeks that my brother and I tramped through those wonderful groves, I can only imagine what a magical childhood Mom must have had.

Slowly Awakening

Mom remained on a ventilator. External signs of change in the early weeks were hard to see. She also had foot drop, which happens when a brain no longer functions.

We listened to arguments between the neurologists and the cardiologists as to the extent of damage and chances of her return. An echocardiogram showed Mom's heart to be all right. They tried to take her off the ventilator several times without success. Finally, the day came when they removed the ventilator and she was able to breathe on her own.

She couldn't talk because she was paralyzed, yet she seemed aware of things. Her eyes, looking around her room, seemed filled with distress. We would tell her, "You have had a stroke, and are just coming out of a coma, but you are getting better." Soon she would communicate by blinking once for yes and twice for no. She could hold her head up slightly, and soon she was beginning to move first one arm, then the other.

When Mom first woke up, we would give her music with headphones. She could indicate whether or not she wanted to listen to music by the blinking. One of the first words she spoke was to her night nurse, Marilyn, who turned off the room lights and said goodnight. Mom responded, "Goodnight, Marilyn." She had made a comment that was appropriate to the conversation. These little signs told us that Mom was still with us.

Then one day while visiting the ICU, two of her co-workers came out of her room in tears. Fearful of those dreaded words, I ran over to one of the women. "What happened, Linda? Is Mom dead?"

Linda slowly sat down with me and said, "Your mom's brain damage looks very bad."

"Why?"

"When the nurse on duty asked if she would like to listen to the radio, your mother spoke some strange words."

"What did she say?"

"Your mother asked to listen to Howard Stern."

Linda must have thought me nuts when I immediately hugged her and proclaimed that Mom was going to be all right. For years Mom had been a closet-fan of Howard Stern. She hid it so well that Linda, who had been in the office next to her for over four years, had no idea that Mom listened to Howard or lesbian-dial-a-date while sipping her nonfat lattes and getting ready for surgery.

If Mom is asking to listen to Howard Stern, it means that she is skipping back from the twilight.

Recovery

First she had to regain her strength from three months being motionless in the ICU so she was transferred to the rehabilitation unit. She had to learn to walk and talk again. She moved from a wheelchair to a walker and eventually to a cane. Now, in less than a year, she can walk without any assistance at all.

She lost a lot of confidence because she couldn't return to work, even though she is still has an alert, intelligent mind. If she feels pressure from anything, she gets anxious like never before. Each year she continues to improve remarkably. She has short-term memory lapses, yet she can to drive. She went to driving school, passed her test, and took a huge step to freedom. She still doesn't drive on the freeway, but she does fine around town.

She stopped listening to Howard Stern. She didn't think he was funny anymore. Instead she called him crass—a sure sign that, although her tastes have changed some, her ability to form a strong opinion has not.

She does yoga to increase strength and flexibility. I believe she attributes yoga to saving her life, in that she could go to a place in her mind and meditate, to relax and find inner peace.

Her ability to relax and find within herself a quiet strength was also extremely important during the painful coming-out process. Learning to walk and talk again, to stretch and learn again to use her body, was distressing. Mom was incredible!

Mom's reunion with the twins was slower since they had grown so much since her first association with them. I took my son and daughter to her while she was in rehabilitation and laid them on the bed where she was sitting. It was awkward because she was afraid they would fall off the bed. Also her body was shaky and she wasn't confident holding them. It took time for her to feel comfortable with them again but eventually their bond became warm and deep.

The children only know her as she is today. They are afraid for her. We might be hiking with one child on a horse, and Mom walking more slowly behind us, and my son will stop and say, "We can't go on ahead because grandma could get lost out here." He seems to have a genuine awareness that she might occasionally need assistance.

What Mom has accomplished is amazing. People do not realize that she ever had a stroke. And she is married to the most patient, wonderful man in the world. My father took over Mom's running of the house, like paying the bills and managing the household tasks. They are continuing their wonderful journey together.

Chapter Eleven

Can Anything More Happen?

> *The question is not whether we will die, but how we will live.*
>
> ~ Joan Borysenko

We were happy to have persevered through the kid's first year. My mom's stroke and my gall bladder surgery were behind us. Our spirits were lifted as we watched Mom's progress.

I was determined to be the best mom I could be. I didn't want to miss any more of my babies' lives so I let our dear nanny go. I was still exhausted, however, and couldn't seem to renew my energy. Despite my recent surgery, I was still periodically jaundiced. My liver enzyme count was high and I was clearly sick, so more medical tests were necessary.

Hepatitis wasn't on top of the doctor's list for my illness. Eventually he did test me for it and I came up positive, so they retested me. I came up positive again. Apparently hepatitis was running rampant in my liver, exacerbated by the pregnancy and the stress of mom's illness.

I was stunned. My first concern was for my children and husband not to contract it. The doctor reassured me that it would be very unlikely that any of them could. He gave them less than a 3% chance of contracting it from me, but we had the three of them tested. Even when the negative test came back, I had them tested again just to be sure. Negative again. I was so relieved.

Hepatitis C is a very lethal disease and frequently thought of as incurable. However, chemotherapy treatments can be successful against certain genotypes. Unfortunately the chemotherapy itself can have severe, adverse affects and is not always recommended.

The doctor who first saw me advised me not to get treatment. I could not accept that recommendation. I could not allow myself to get sick. I was not going to allow myself to die of liver failure and leave my kids without a mother. I left the doctors office resolved to do my own research.

Armed with increased knowledge, I returned and confronted the doctor. "You don't even know what genotype I have. How can you say that treatments only have a fifty percent cure rate you don't even know my virus's genotype? One genotype has a cure rate of 80 to 90 percent. "

He said, "Well, you won't have that type."

"You don't know that, and it is your job to find out for me." I pushed the issue, "You have to find out for me." The doctor finally agreed to check the genotype and cure rates of treatment. If I were not my own advocate, what would have happened?

This was a good doctor but he wasn't going to be my advocate. He wasn't pushing for a treatment that he knew might have serious side affects and only a fifty percent chance of actually working. But it wasn't his choice to make. It was mine.

I went to the lab and got my hepatitis virus genotyped. It turned out I had a rare strain of hepatitis C-2A, which is found mostly in Asia and uncommon in the United States. My doctors and I scoured my past to determine where I could have picked it up. In the 1980s, as acupuncture was gaining popularity in the United States, my mother took me to Asian acupuncturists for everything from nail biting and bad knees to sports injuries and stress. Not only was I the only kid I ever saw there, I was the only Caucasian girl. Back then people used needles without sterilization. That is my theory anyway and it gave me an answer to how I contracted it.

With the genotype identified, I proceeded to another doctor at to get a second opinion. In conversation with the new doctor, I discovered that he had attended medical school with my first doctor. He said, "Well, this is insane. You should do this treatment. You've got an incredibly curable genotype and I'm going to recommend to your doctor that you should go ahead and do the treatment."

The first doctor backpedaled quickly. "Well I didn't know, of course, I think you should get the treatment."

Finally! I was getting some action.

I needed to start a chemotherapy treatment right away before the hepatitis did even more damage to my liver and then other organs. The doctors told me how difficult the treatments would be and that I should consider getting some help with the kids. I was determined to start the treatments on my own and see how I felt.

Treatment

When the treatment began with the first injection of interferon, I was shaking with fear. Two nurses were present in case I went into anaphylactic shock any time during the twenty minutes that the stuff was moving through my body. Hey, twenty minutes passed and I was still awake and well. Next, they injected the second batch and we waited again. Do you know how slow twenty minutes feels when two nurses are waiting for you to keel over?

Nothing adverse happened. I was fine. I continued the regimen. Each day I swallowed a handful of pills. Each week, my husband administered a shot to my abdomen. We joked that he was back to giving me shots like he did during my IVF process.

The first two months of treatment didn't seem too bad. Unfortunately, I did experience one of the difficult aspects of having an illness like Hepatitis C, especially a rare strain. I had to deal with people's ignorance. A typical example was when one of the nurses who treated me also lectured me during treatment. "Well, if you do risky behaviors…" and "Hopefully, you won't get it again, but if you go out there and do that stuff…"

I finally hissed, "What are you talking about?"

"You know, drugs, tattoos, that kind of stuff."

Now I was livid. "You know, first of all, you don't know who I am. Second of all, don't blame the victim," which is exactly what she was doing. She was a pretty negative and prejudicial person to be in that position of treating patients.

Occasionally, a doctor might say, "Oh well, you know you did this to yourself. You brought this onto yourself." Yeah right, Doc! I can't even imagine how people with HIV would feel if treated with such remarks. Hepatitis C can be a fatal disease if it's not treated. Your liver might eventually fail. The disease is bad enough without medical professionals laying guilt trips on ill people.

Fortunately, they did blood work on me every four weeks. By week eight, the disease was gone. I was ecstatic. Tired but ecstatic. I still had four months of treatments left, but it was working. I would be completely cured.

My seemingly smooth ride ended by month three. I started to go downhill. My thick, Irish, curly, reddish-blonde hair started thinning out, although I did not lose it, thank heavens. I did drop some post-pregnancy weight and the additional twenty pounds of "stress" food I had eaten after my mom's illness. I think that was the only positive part.

I was exhausted, really wiped out from the tiniest of efforts. A few days of the week I would force myself out of bed and take the twins to the local YMCA, which has a wonderful childcare facility. I would stretch my time to two hours by riding the exercise bike while watching television, soaking in the Jacuzzi or steaming up a hot shower. I wasn't trying to get in great shape. My goal was to keep my circulation going.

The last four weeks were the hardest. I was so drained but I knew I had to ride out the treatments to the end to guarantee that the hepatitis would not return. I told myself that there were things much worse than the treatments, like not being around to raise my children. I had so much to live for. I couldn't imagine not raising my children, not being there for them. I did not let any other outcome play in my mind. I focused only on one goal: I was going to be cured. I was going to make it through this. That was it. I refused to entertain any ideas about death or failure.

Finally, the treatments were over and I was given a clean bill of health.

More Drama

I went back to my insurance company as soon as I was done. I said, "You know what, I'm cured now, do a blood test on me. I want to get more life insurance." I was getting my life in order.

They did the blood work. My regular insurance agent was out of town and his wife was running the office. She didn't even call me back. Her secretary called and said, "Oh you've been denied."

My heart sunk. "Excuse me?" I asked in a whisper.

"Oh, they said you still have it. So sorry, we can't help you."

I was stunned. I thought, oh my God, it's come back. I've

done all this blood work, all these treatments, and they said, without a doubt, you're completely cured. I slipped into hysterics. I was at work so I walked out into the parking lot, sat down and sobbed. I called the clinic. A nurse answered and I told her what happened: "My insurance company said I'm not cured. I don't know what to do. I'm just so upset, you know. You guys said I was okay and they're saying I'm not."

"You know, those people, they just did the sensitivity test which showed you had sensitivity. You have no levels. You're fine. Don't worry about it. Okay. I've got to go." And she hung up on me.

I became more hysterical. She just didn't give me any time to find out what to do next, so I called my family practice doctor who happened to be out. I hopped in my car and drove to the clinic. I saw a different doctor.

"You need to do a levels test for me to show that my levels are completely gone" I demanded. He put a rush on it for me. When the results indicated that I was clear of hepatitis, he wrote me a letter testifying that I'm completely cured and that it would never return. He stated that I was completely healthy and listed my levels to prove it.

Later that same day, a nursing supervisor called me and asked me if I had talked to nurse so and so.

"Yes, I did. You know I was going make a phone call actually to report her. This was going to be the second time I'd made a report about her because she was so horrible to me."

"She told me of the conversation she had with you. I was so horrified by her behavior and how she responded to you. I'm her supervisor and I wanted to make sure you were okay."

"You know, I'm very upset today, and these test results really scared me."

She was calm as she talked to me; "I'm going to take action on this."

I don't know whatever happened to that nurse, but I'm so glad someone didn't let her continue to treat patients so rudely.

In all that I went through, that was the only time I ever broke down tearfully and lost it.

I needed to find a new insurance agent. There was no way I was going to continue to do business with an agent that would not fight for me. I decided that I wanted a strong woman to represent me. I interviewed two women with the same agency. One woman stepped to the fore: "You know what? I've never had anything like this, but you have a case here. I'm sending this to the front office and there's no reason why they'll deny it." Later she mentioned that she thought I was the first person to have ever been treated with Hepatitis C and get full life insurance. My agent is an amazing woman and I am grateful that she went to bat for me.

If you are ever gravely ill, fight to find the right people to get in your corner. I was completely healthy but they still wanted to label my health as uncertain for the rest of my life. I was ready to put up a fight and I was fortunate to find someone who was willing to fight with me.

Chapter Twelve

The Fighting Spirit

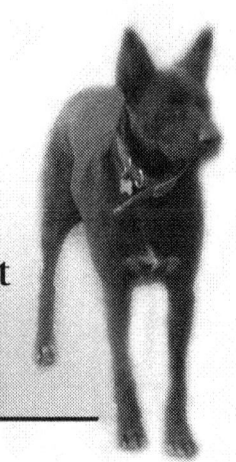

Immediately following my treatments, I didn't talk about my illness. After my gall bladder surgery, my mom almost dying and my Hepatitis C situation, I couldn't bring myself to open up anymore. Not only was I dealing with the prejudice within the medical community, but also I hate people feeling sorry for me. I cringe when I think of people saying, "Oh, poor Jenn."

I think I have a problem with that because I've been a real fighter my whole life. I've had to because of my learning disability. People were always coming down on me; I can think of so many instances in my life where people were telling me not to move forward because there's no point.

I was belittled when at a young age I went to a center for people with learning disabilities, seeking help in finding an appropriate college. I had found information on Landmark College and showed this to the center's director.

"What do you think of this place? Do you know anything about it?" I asked.

She looked at me so sincerely and responded, "I need to be perfectly frank with you. You are so severely dyslexic that this would be a terrible waste of your parents' money. I think you should go to beautician school."

"What? You know, I can't even do my own hair. I can't. I have nothing against beauticians but there's no way. I want to go to college. I want a formal education. I've never received one and I have to have this."

"Well don't go to Landmark. It is too expensive, and it would waste your parents' money."

Fortunately I did not take her advice and I went to Landmark. If not for the outstanding education I received there, I would have never gone on to receive my bachelor's degree from a four-year college. Am I sensitive to prejudice and injustice based on ignorance? You bet I am.

Thank heavens both of my parents and my brother believed in me. Even when I announced that I was dropping out of high school and moving to Europe at age seventeen, they understood I needed a break from education and a look at real life. Hey, they probably needed a break from me too!

I couldn't sit in a classroom and understand what was

happening. I was intimidated, frustrated and sad. I remember when the faculty tried to place me in "mainstream education" during my freshman year in high school. I went to class for four hours in the morning with a bunch of immature boys who were always in trouble. In the afternoon I was a standout varsity gymnast and diver. So they locked me away in the gym the rest of the day.

There wasn't an effective learning-disabled program in my school at that time. By law, the school had to pay for the child's education and find the best education if they couldn't provide it and they couldn't for me. The school officials told my parents and me that we could fight for it but it would take years and I would be in my twenties. School officials intimidated us into leaving it alone.

By my sophomore year, I was fifteen-years old, taking mainstream classes, and reading and writing at a fourth-grade level. It is horrible trying to be like everyone else when you're not. It is even harder when you are a fifteen-year-old girl.

Besides the people at Landmark, one of the only educators who was ever in my corner was my Menlo College advisor, the school I transferred to after Landmark. I blessed his soul as he died two years ago. I still think of him with gratitude. He was somebody who believed in me. He saw that I could write and he knew that I was intelligent; I was just having a hard time expressing myself. He talked to my other professors in philosophy and art history about dyslexia. A few professors were well into their sixties and knew nothing of learning disabilities or how to help students learn new information. Yet, I told them both that I had to take my tests un-timed.

A few of them said no one had ever done that and they weren't going to start. At that time a girl from UC Berkley had just sued Berkley because they wouldn't let her do it. I carried that article around with me, and I gave copies to both of them and said, "I will sue this school if you don't do this." One professor stayed pissed off at me the whole semester. He just gave me Bs with no references to my papers. The other professor researched the law and the topic and made it his business to learn about dyslexia. He took his time and showed interest in my work. Yes, I've had to fight for my rights every step of the way.

What if I had listened to everyone else except my parents and myself? What if I had not fought? I couldn't imagine what kind of a person I would be. I wouldn't have finished school. I would have walked away from it many years ago. Just imagine, I could be childless, riddled with Hepatitis C and doing really bad hair jobs on people.

A philosophy professor of mine once gave us an assignment to pick out a song that identified who we were. The song

I picked was, Jimmy Cliff's "The Harder They Come," the soundtrack for the movie by the same name. The movie depicted the story of a Kingston (Jamaica) reggae singer who became a modern Robin Hood. The harder they tried to keep him down, the harder he fought.

We all have things to fight for. Cancer survivors need to keep a fighting spirit to get through their treatments, as do many others with potentially fatal illnesses. When I wanted to give up my hepatitis treatments, I would think of my children and gather the strength to go on. Thinking of them help me always put my life into perspective.

Chapter Thirteen

Blessed

Harold: Maude.
Maude: Hmm?
Harold: Do you pray?
Maude: Pray? No. I communicate.
Harold: With God?
Maude: With *life*.

Harold and Maude, 1971

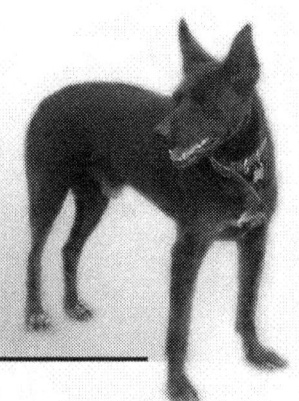

As we were driving home from dinner several weeks ago, my five-year old son broke the silence to ask us, "Is God a real person or an actor"? After my husband stopped his tear-filled laughter, Robert looked at me and asked again, "Well, who is this God that your son is asking about"? I loved how he put me on the spot to give a good, truthful and meaningful explanation as to what or who God is.

Just yesterday I told Robert that I read this quote about

book promotion: "Once you write a book on a subject, you have now become an expert on the subject." I certainly feel like an expert on resilience, but I sure have had a hard time explaining God to my son.

I have spent a lifetime with such conflicting feelings about God and his/her/its existence, that even if I earned a PhD in theology, I would still not be an expert on God.

I turned to my children in the backseat and calmly explained that many people in the world believe that God create the Earth and everything in it.

My daughter looked at her brother and said convincingly, "Yes, God made everything—like cars."

To which he queried in all seriousness, "and potties?" She said, "Yes, potties too." So much for our first attempt on the subject of theology.

Robert, unlike me, grew up spending his Sundays at a Catholic Mass. He went through his first communion and confirmation. But, like so many of the other Catholics in my life, he had jumped off the religion wagon a long time ago. So Robert enjoyed the God-made-the-potty giggles of the children. However, I wanted to be better prepared the next time the topic was raised. As soon as we put the kids to bed that night, I did what any modern woman would do. I went online and ordered four books on explaining God and religion to children. And I ordered one on death and dying even though that topic had not come up yet. I wanted to be prepared.

Since my children have come into my life, I am finally heeding my father's advice. I walk much slower now and not just because they have to stop and look at everything. One Saturday, Dad and I put the kids on one of their older horses, a former wild stallion that is now the kids' horse who takes them for walks in the park. We walked out along the park next to my parent's property. We took a long walk and we counted all the animals. Without the children, I wouldn't have noticed so many butterflies. We counted six dragonflies.

In the middle of our walk, my son started screaming, "Grandpa! Stop! Stop!" In the distant bushes he spied a baby doe. He was so proud of himself for seeing it.

Then my daughter said, "There's a gopher. Or maybe it's a rabbit." Then my son yells, "It's a gopher in a rabbit's outfit because it's almost Halloween."

The children laugh so freely that I find myself doing the same. They have a great sense of humor. They offer, and I return, the most amazing unconditional love that I've ever felt.

So how can we begin to understand God, who is defined in so many different ways by so many different religions?

Reflecting back on my roller coast ride of the past five years, this is what I think:

Focus on the same core message that most religions teach:

help those who are in need of help;

be truthful;

do not harm others; and

do not take what is not yours.

Most of all, appreciate whatever you have—feel blessed:

I feel blessed when I walk to the top of my favorite hiking trail and look out over the San Francisco Bay Area on a clear day.

I feel blessed by my family's sense of togetherness and perseverance.

I feel blessed whenever my children laugh.

I feel blessed by my dog's grateful lick after a long walk.

I feel blessed when I recognize joy in the middle of an awful day.

I feel blessed when I am able to bring food to a homeless shelter with my children.

I feel blessed when my husband's love shines through his eyes when he looks at me.

I feel blessed when I connect with God.

For me, it is not formal praying that connects me to God. I feel connected to God when I see all those who are blessed around me. I feel the presence of God whenever I think about how blessed I am. That connection makes me feel blessed. That is the connection that enables me to radiate the love and hope I feel everyday.

My greatest role now is now caring for my children. I want to teach them how they can be moral and good. I want them to feel as blessed as I do everyday. I want to help them find that divine spark that lies within all of us, that lies within them and show them how to let it shine.

Publishing the Works of Extraordinary Mom Writers

Wyatt-MacKenzie Publishing, Inc

WyMacPublishing.com

www.ingramcontent.com/pod-product-compliance
Lightning Source LLC
LaVergne TN
LVHW091311080426
835510LV00007B/472